I0765358

GASTRIC BYPASS

COOKBOOK

FOR ALL STAGES

Easy and Healthy Recipes to Eat Well after Weight Loss Surgery

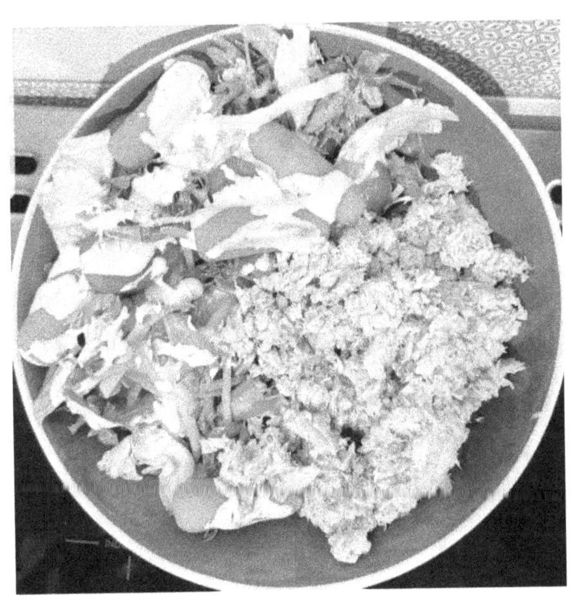

DR. RICHARDSON DAVIDS

COPYRIGHT 2024

All right reserved

No part of this book may be produced or transmitted in any form whatsoever, electronic, or mechanical including photocopying, recording or by any informational storage and retrieval system without the express written, dated and signed permission of the Author.

TABLE OF CONTENTS

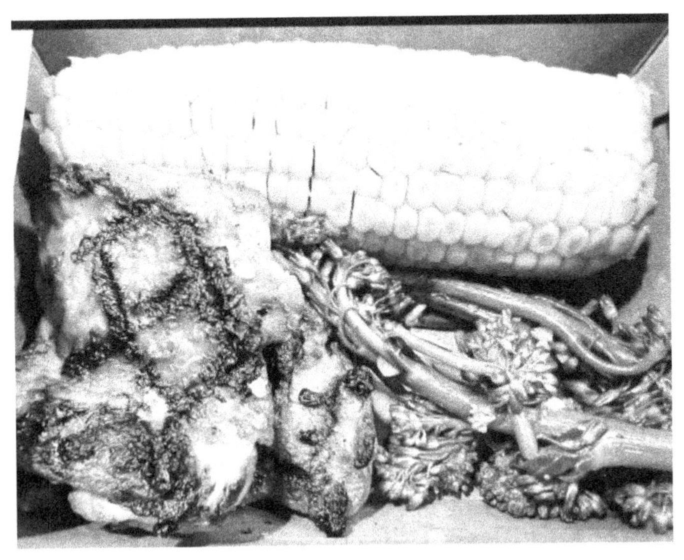

INTRODUCTION

Achieving a healthier and more fulfilling life is a major step before beginning the life-changing procedure of gastric bypass surgery. However, the post-operative recovery phase presents unique challenges, particularly with regard to maintaining a nutritious and well-balanced diet. This cookbook is meant to serve as your go-to source for a wide range of delicious and nutritious recipes that will assist you in meeting your dietary needs after gastric bypass surgery.

The digestive tract is altered after gastric bypass surgery, thus cautious food selection is now required. Regardless of how much experience you have with bypass surgery, this cookbook is customized to fit your specific requirements. Each recipe has been carefully selected to meet both your post-surgery nutritional demands and your desire for a satisfying dinner.

Within these pages, you'll find a variety of delicious dishes catered to the specific dietary requirements and preferences of gastric bypass patients. We've developed a broad variety of foods, from nutrient-dense snacks to protein-rich dinners, that strike a balance between taste and nutrition. We want to help you create a positive and long-lasting eating habit and a positive relationship with food to complement your newly found health path.

We also understand that recovering from a gastric bypass can be challenging, and the last thing you need is additional anxiety in the kitchen. Because of this, each dish is designed to be easy to follow, using readily available ingredients and straightforward directions, allowing meal preparation to become a part of your daily routine.

As you navigate this culinary adventure, let our Gastric Bypass Cookbook serve as your go-to resource for creating meals that uplift your spirit and body. Cheers to savoring every bite on your path to becoming a more positive, healthier version of yourself.

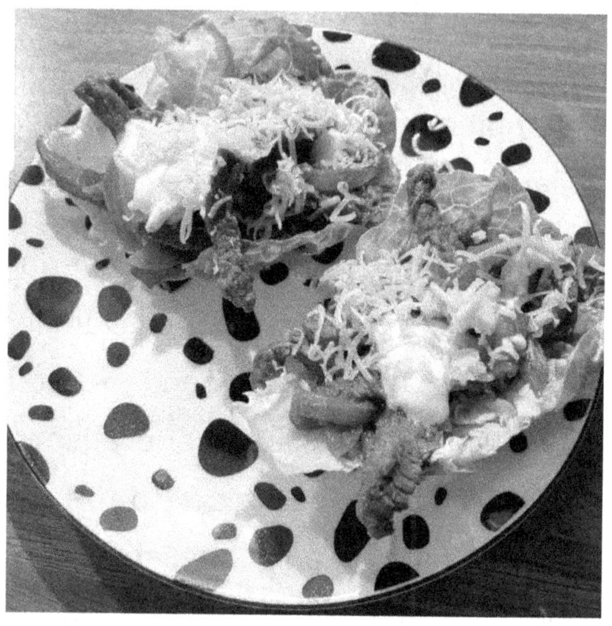

BREAKFAST

PROTEIN-PACKED OMELETTE

Cooking Time: 10 minutes

Nutritional Benefits: High protein content for sustained energy.

Ingredients:

2 large eggs

1/4 cup diced turkey or chicken

1/4 cup chopped spinach

Salt and pepper to taste

Method:

Whisk eggs and pour into a hot, non-stick pan.

Add turkey, spinach, salt, and pepper.

Cook until eggs are set.

GREEK YOGURT PARFAIT

Cooking Time: 5 minutes

Nutritional Benefits: Rich in protein and probiotics for digestive health.

Ingredients:

1/2 cup Greek yogurt

1/4 cup berries (strawberries, blueberries)

2 tablespoons granola

1 tablespoon honey

Method:

Layer yogurt, berries, and granola.

Drizzle honey on top.

SPINACH AND FETA FRITTATA CUPS

Cooking Time: 15 minutes

Nutritional Benefits: Packed with vitamins and minerals from spinach and protein from eggs.

Ingredients:

4 eggs

1/2 cup chopped spinach

1/4 cup crumbled feta cheese

Salt and pepper to taste

Method:

Mix eggs, spinach, feta, salt, and pepper.

Pour into muffin tin and bake until set.

QUINOA BREAKFAST BOWL

Cooking Time: 5 minutes

Nutritional Benefits: Quinoa provides a complete protein source, and chia seeds add omega-3 fatty acids.

Ingredients:

1/2 cup cooked quinoa

1/4 cup almond milk

1/4 cup sliced bananas

1 tablespoon chia seeds

Method:

Mix quinoa, almond milk, bananas, and chia seeds.

COTTAGE CHEESE AND PINEAPPLE SALAD

Cooking Time: 5 minutes

Nutritional Benefits: Cottage cheese offers a protein boost, and pineapple provides vitamins and natural sweetness.

Ingredients:

1/2 cup low-fat cottage cheese

1/2 cup fresh pineapple chunks

1 tablespoon chopped mint

Method:

Combine cottage cheese, pineapple, and mint.

SMOOTHIE BOWL

Preparation Time: 7 minutes

Nutritional Benefits: Packed with antioxidants, fiber, and protein for a nutritious and delicious start.

Ingredients:

1/2 cup unsweetened almond milk

1/2 cup frozen mixed berries

1/2 banana, sliced

1 scoop protein powder

Method:

Blend almond milk, berries, banana, and protein powder.

Pour into a bowl and add toppings of choice.

SALMON AND AVOCADO TOAST

Preparation Time: 8 minutes

Nutritional Benefits: Omega-3 fatty acids from salmon and healthy fats from avocado.

Ingredients:

2 oz smoked salmon

1/2 avocado, mashed

1 slice whole-grain toast

Lemon wedge

Method:

Spread mashed avocado on toast.

Top with smoked salmon and a squeeze of lemon.

EGG MUFFIN CUPS

Cooking Time: 15 minutes

Nutritional Benefits: High protein and low-carb option with added veggies.

Ingredients:

4 eggs

1/4 cup diced bell peppers

1/4 cup diced turkey sausage

Salt and pepper to taste

Method:

Whisk eggs, add peppers, turkey sausage, salt, and pepper.

Pour into muffin tin and bake until set.

CHIA SEED PUDDING

Preparation Time: 5 minutes (plus overnight chilling)

Nutritional Benefits: Rich in omega-3s, fiber, and antioxidants.

Ingredients:

2 tablespoons chia seeds

1/2 cup unsweetened almond milk

1/4 teaspoon vanilla extract

Fresh berries for topping

Method:

Mix chia seeds, almond milk, and vanilla. Refrigerate overnight.

Top with fresh berries before serving.

TURKEY AND VEGETABLE SCRAMBLE

Cooking Time: 12 minutes

Nutritional Benefits: Lean protein from turkey and a variety of veggies for added nutrients.

Ingredients:

1/2 cup ground turkey, cooked

1/4 cup diced zucchini

1/4 cup cherry tomatoes, halved

2 eggs, beaten

Method:

Cook turkey, add zucchini and tomatoes.

Pour in beaten eggs, scramble until cooked.

BANANA AND ALMOND BUTTER TOAST

Preparation Time: 5 minutes

Nutritional Benefits: Provides healthy fats, protein, and natural sweetness.

Ingredients:

1 slice whole-grain bread

1 tablespoon almond butter

1/2 banana, sliced

Method:

Toast the bread and spread almond butter.

Top with banana slices.

MUSHROOM AND SPINACH EGG WRAP

Cooking Time: 8 minutes

Nutritional Benefits: High in protein and vitamins from eggs and veggies.

Ingredients:

2 large eggs

1/4 cup sliced mushrooms

1/2 cup fresh spinach

Whole-grain tortilla

Method:

Scramble eggs, sauté mushrooms and spinach.

Fill tortilla with the mixture.

RICOTTA AND BERRY STUFFED CREPES

Preparation Time: 10 minutes

Nutritional Benefits: Protein-rich and packed with antioxidants.

Ingredients:

2 whole-grain crepes

1/2 cup low-fat ricotta cheese

Mixed berries for stuffing

Method:

Spread ricotta on crepes, add mixed berries.

Fold and serve.

SWEET POTATO HASH WITH EGG

Cooking Time: 12 minutes

Nutritional Benefits: Vitamin A from sweet potatoes and protein from the egg.

Ingredients:

1/2 cup sweet potato, grated

1/4 cup diced bell peppers

1 egg

1 teaspoon olive oil

Method:

Sauté sweet potato and bell peppers in olive oil.

Create a well, crack an egg, and cook until the egg is set.

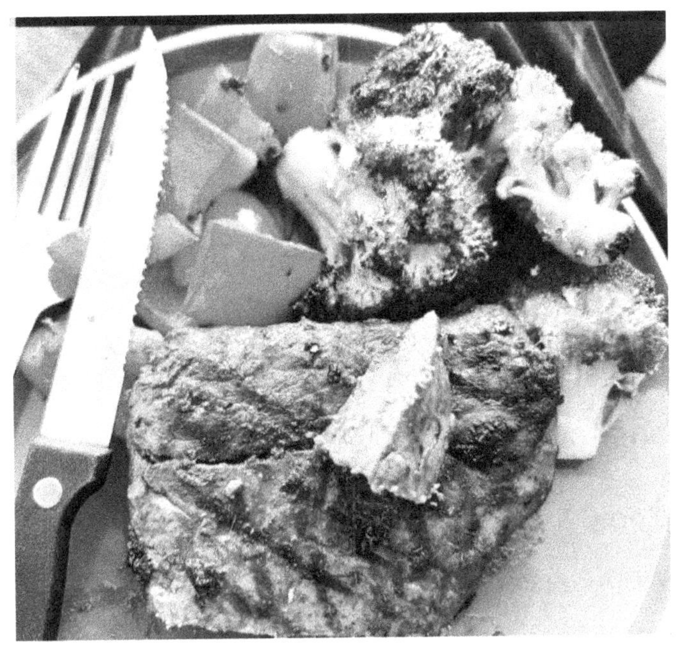

GREEK OMELETTE WRAP

Cooking Time: 10 minutes

Nutritional Benefits: Protein-packed with a Mediterranean flair.

Ingredients:

2 large eggs

1/4 cup diced tomatoes

1/4 cup chopped cucumbers

1 tablespoon feta cheese

Whole-grain wrap

Method:

Whisk eggs, add tomatoes, cucumbers, and feta.

Cook into an omelette, then wrap in a whole-grain tortilla.

AVOCADO AND EGG SALAD

Preparation Time: 7 minutes

Nutritional Benefits: Healthy fats from avocado and protein from egg.

Ingredients:

1 boiled egg, chopped

1/2 avocado, mashed

1 teaspoon Dijon mustard

Salt and pepper to taste

Method:

Mix chopped egg, mashed avocado, mustard, salt, and pepper.

Spread on whole-grain toast.

APPLE CINNAMON QUINOA PORRIDGE

Cooking Time: 5 minutes

Nutritional Benefits: Quinoa provides protein, and apples add fiber and natural sweetness.

Ingredients:

1/2 cup cooked quinoa

1/2 apple, grated

1/4 teaspoon cinnamon

1 tablespoon chopped nuts (almonds or walnuts)

Mix quinoa, grated apple, cinnamon, and top with chopped nuts.

COTTAGE CHEESE AND STRAWBERRY WRAP

Preparation Time: 5 minutes

Nutritional Benefits: High protein and vitamin C from cottage cheese and strawberries.

Ingredients:

1/2 cup low-fat cottage cheese

1/2 cup sliced strawberries

Whole-grain wrap

Method:

Spread cottage cheese on the wrap, add sliced strawberries.

Roll it up and enjoy.

TOMATO AND MOZZARELLA EGG CUPS

Cooking Time: 10 minutes

Nutritional Benefits: Protein and lycopene-rich breakfast option.

Ingredients:

2 eggs

1/2 cup cherry tomatoes, halved

1/4 cup mozzarella cheese, shredded

Fresh basil leaves for garnish

Crack eggs into muffin tin, add tomatoes and mozzarella.

Bake until eggs are set, garnish with basil.

CHICKEN SAUSAGE AND VEGGIE SKILLET

Cooking Time: 12 minutes

Nutritional Benefits: Lean protein from chicken sausage and a mix of veggies for added nutrients.

Ingredients:

1 chicken sausage, sliced

1/2 cup diced bell peppers

1/4 cup diced onions

2 eggs

Sauté sausage, bell peppers, and onions in a skillet.

Add eggs and cook until done.

SPICED CHIA PUDDING

Preparation Time: 5 minutes (plus chilling time)

Nutritional Benefits: Chia seeds provide omega-3s, and kiwi adds vitamin C.

Ingredients:

2 tablespoons chia seeds

1/2 cup unsweetened almond milk

1/4 teaspoon cinnamon

1/4 teaspoon nutmeg

Sliced kiwi for topping

Method:

Mix chia seeds, almond milk, cinnamon, and nutmeg. Refrigerate until thickened.

Top with sliced kiwi before serving.

HAM AND CHEESE EGG MUFFINS

Cooking Time: 15 minutes

Nutritional Benefits: Protein-packed with the goodness of ham and cheese.

Ingredients:

4 eggs

1/4 cup diced ham

1/4 cup shredded cheddar cheese

Salt and pepper to taste

Method:

Whisk eggs, add ham, cheese, salt, and pepper.

Pour into muffin tin and bake until set.

TURMERIC SCRAMBLED EGGS

Cooking Time: 8 minutes

Nutritional Benefits: Anti-inflammatory properties from turmeric and a boost of protein.

Ingredients:

3 eggs

1/4 teaspoon turmeric

1/4 cup diced tomatoes

Fresh cilantro for garnish

Whisk eggs, add turmeric, and diced tomatoes.

Cook until eggs are scrambled, garnish with cilantro.

BERRY AND ALMOND SMOOTHIE

Preparation Time: 5 minutes

Nutritional Benefits: Antioxidants from berries and protein from almond butter and powder.

Ingredients:

1/2 cup mixed berries (strawberries, blueberries, raspberries)

1/2 cup unsweetened almond milk

1 scoop vanilla protein powder

1 tablespoon almond butter

Blend berries, almond milk, protein powder, and almond butter until smooth.

CAPRESE AVOCADO TOAST

Preparation Time: 7 minutes
Nutritional Benefits: Healthy fats from avocado and antioxidants from tomatoes and basil.

Ingredients:

1 slice whole-grain bread

1/2 avocado, mashed

1/2 cup cherry tomatoes, sliced

Fresh basil leaves for garnish

Toast the bread, spread mashed avocado, top with sliced tomatoes, and garnish with basil.

SWEET POTATO PANCAKES

Cooking Time: 10 minutes

Nutritional Benefits: Sweet potatoes provide vitamins and fiber, and eggs add protein.

Ingredients:

1/2 cup mashed sweet potato

2 eggs

1/4 teaspoon cinnamon

1/4 teaspoon vanilla extract

Mix mashed sweet potato, eggs, cinnamon, and vanilla.

Cook pancakes on a griddle until golden brown.

CHICKEN AND VEGETABLE BREAKFAST STIR-FRY

Cooking Time: 12 minutes

Nutritional Benefits: High protein and a variety of veggies for essential nutrients.

Ingredients:

1/2 cup cooked chicken, shredded

1/2 cup broccoli florets

1/4 cup sliced bell peppers

2 eggs

Method:

Sauté chicken, broccoli, and bell peppers in a pan.

Add eggs and stir until cooked.

ALMOND FLOUR WAFFLES

Cooking Time: 15 minutes

Nutritional Benefits: Almond flour provides a gluten-free alternative with healthy fats.

Ingredients:

1 cup almond flour

2 eggs

1/2 cup almond milk

1/2 teaspoon baking powder

Method:

Mix almond flour, eggs, almond milk, and baking powder.

Pour into a waffle maker and cook until golden.

TURKEY BACON AND EGG CUPS

Cooking Time: 12 minutes

Nutritional Benefits: Lean protein from turkey bacon and eggs.

Ingredients:

4 eggs

4 slices turkey bacon

Salt and pepper to taste

Method:

Line muffin tin with turkey bacon.

Crack an egg into each cup, season, and bake until eggs are set.

MANGO COCONUT CHIA SMOOTHIE BOWL

Preparation Time: 7 minutes

Nutritional Benefits: Rich in fiber, healthy fats, and vitamins from mango and coconut.

Ingredients:

1/2 cup diced mango

1/2 cup coconut milk

2 tablespoons chia seeds

Toppings: shredded coconut, sliced almonds

Method:

Blend mango, coconut milk, and chia seeds.

Pour into a bowl, add toppings.

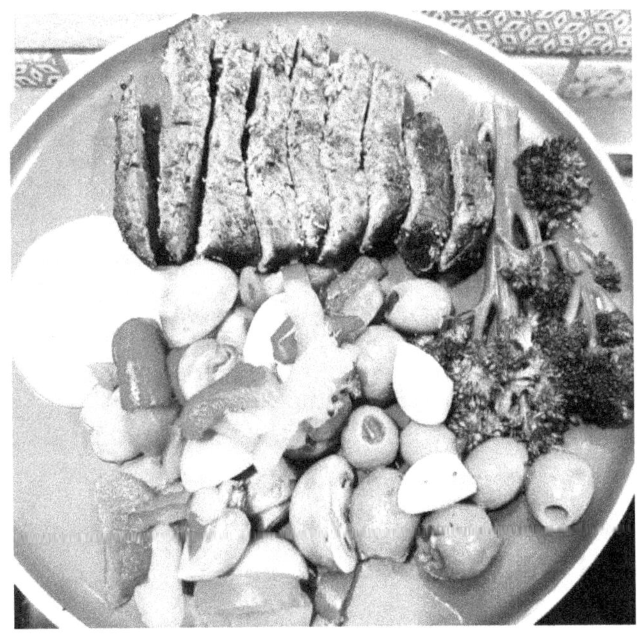

LUNCH

GRILLED CHICKEN SALAD
WITH AVOCADO DRESSING

Preparation Time: 15 minutes

Nutritional Benefits: Lean protein from chicken, healthy fats from avocado, and antioxidants from greens.

Ingredients:

4 oz grilled chicken breast

2 cups mixed greens

1/2 avocado, mashed

1 tablespoon olive oil

1 tablespoon balsamic vinegar

Method:

Combine grilled chicken and mixed greens.

Whisk mashed avocado, olive oil, and balsamic vinegar for dressing.

QUINOA AND VEGETABLE STUFFED PEPPERS

Cooking Time: 25 minutes

Nutritional Benefits: Quinoa provides complete protein, and veggies offer vitamins and fiber.

Ingredients:

1/2 cup cooked quinoa

2 bell peppers, halved

1/4 cup black beans

1/4 cup diced tomatoes

1/4 cup shredded cheese

Mix quinoa, black beans, tomatoes, and stuff into bell peppers.

Sprinkle shredded cheese on top and bake until peppers are tender.

TURKEY AND VEGGIE LETTUCE WRAPS

Preparation Time: 20 minutes

Nutritional Benefits: Lean protein from turkey and a low-carb, veggie-packed option.

Ingredients:

4 oz ground turkey, cooked

Large lettuce leaves

1/4 cup diced bell peppers

1/4 cup shredded carrots

1 tablespoon hoisin sauce

Method:

Fill lettuce leaves with cooked turkey, bell peppers, and carrots.

Drizzle hoisin sauce over the top.

SALMON AND BROCCOLI QUICHE

Cooking Time: 30 minutes

Nutritional Benefits: Omega-3 fatty acids from salmon and essential nutrients from broccoli.

Ingredients:

4 oz cooked salmon, flaked

1 cup broccoli florets

3 eggs

1/2 cup almond milk

Salt and pepper to taste

Method:

Mix salmon and broccoli, pour into a pie dish.

Whisk eggs, almond milk, salt, and pepper, then pour over salmon and broccoli.

Bake until set.

EGG DROP SOUP WITH SPINACH

Cooking Time: 10 minutes

Nutritional Benefits: Protein from eggs and nutrient-rich spinach in a low-calorie soup.

Ingredients:

2 cups chicken broth

2 eggs, beaten

1 cup fresh spinach

1/2 teaspoon ginger, grated

1 tablespoon soy sauce

Method:

Bring chicken broth to a simmer, add ginger and soy sauce.

Slowly pour beaten eggs while stirring.

Add fresh spinach and simmer until wilted.

SHRIMP AND ZOODLE STIR-FRY

Preparation Time: 15 minutes

Nutritional Benefits: Low-calorie and high-protein option with a variety of veggies.

Ingredients:

4 oz shrimp, peeled and deveined

1 zucchini, spiralized

1/4 cup bell peppers, thinly sliced

1 tablespoon sesame oil

1 tablespoon low-sodium soy sauce

Method:

Sauté shrimp, zoodles, and bell peppers in sesame oil.

Drizzle with soy sauce before serving.

TURKEY LETTUCE WRAPS WITH CABBAGE SLAW

Preparation Time: 20 minutes
Nutritional Benefits: Lean protein from turkey and a low-carb, crunchy slaw.

Ingredients:

4 oz ground turkey, cooked

Large cabbage leaves

1/4 cup shredded cabbage

1/4 cup julienned carrots

1 tablespoon Greek yogurt

Method:

Fill cabbage leaves with cooked turkey.

Toss shredded cabbage and carrots with Greek yogurt for slaw.

CHICKEN AND BROCCOLI CASSEROLE

Cooking Time: 25 minutes

Nutritional Benefits: High protein and calcium from chicken and cottage cheese.

Ingredients:

4 oz cooked chicken breast, shredded

1 cup broccoli florets

1/2 cup cottage cheese

1/4 cup grated Parmesan cheese

Salt and pepper to taste

Method:

Mix chicken, broccoli, cottage cheese, and Parmesan.

Bake until bubbly and golden.

MEXICAN CAULIFLOWER RICE BOWL

Preparation Time: 15 minutes

Nutritional Benefits: Low-carb alternative with fiber from cauliflower and healthy fats from avocado.

Ingredients:

1 cup cauliflower rice, cooked

1/4 cup black beans

1/4 cup diced tomatoes

1/4 cup diced avocado

1 tablespoon salsa

Method:

Mix cauliflower rice with black beans, tomatoes, and top with avocado.

Drizzle salsa over the bowl.

VEGETARIAN STUFFED PEPPER SOUP

Cooking Time: 20 minutes

Nutritional Benefits: Low-calorie and rich in vitamins and antioxidants.

Ingredients:

2 bell peppers, diced

1 cup cauliflower rice

2 cups vegetable broth

1/2 cup diced tomatoes

1/4 cup chopped parsley

Method:

Simmer bell peppers, cauliflower rice, vegetable broth, and tomatoes until peppers are tender.

Garnish with chopped parsley before serving.

GREEK CHICKEN SALAD WRAP

Preparation Time: 15 minutes

Nutritional Benefits: Protein-packed with a Mediterranean twist.

Ingredients:

4 oz grilled chicken breast, sliced

Whole-grain wrap

1/4 cup cherry tomatoes, halved

1/4 cup cucumber, diced

2 tablespoons feta cheese

Method:

Fill the wrap with sliced grilled chicken, tomatoes, cucumber, and feta.

Roll it up and enjoy.

CAULIFLOWER CRUST PIZZA

Cooking Time: 25 minutes

Nutritional Benefits: Low-carb pizza alternative with veggies.

Ingredients:

1 cup cauliflower rice

1 egg

1/4 cup tomato sauce

1/4 cup mozzarella cheese

Toppings of choice (spinach, mushrooms, bell peppers)

Method:

Mix cauliflower rice and egg, spread onto a baking sheet.

Bake until golden, add tomato sauce, cheese, and toppings.

Bake until cheese melts.

LEMON GARLIC SHRIMP AND ZUCCHINI NOODLES

Preparation Time: 15 minutes

Nutritional Benefits: Low-calorie, high-protein, and rich in vitamins.

Ingredients:

4 oz shrimp, peeled and deveined

1 zucchini, spiralized

1 tablespoon olive oil

1 clove garlic, minced

1 tablespoon lemon juice

Method:

Sauté shrimp, zoodles, and garlic in olive oil.

Drizzle with lemon juice before serving.

TUNA STUFFED AVOCADO

Preparation Time: 10 minutes

Nutritional Benefits: Omega-3s from tuna and healthy fats from avocado.

Ingredients:

1 can (5 oz) tuna, drained

1/2 avocado, mashed

1/4 cup cherry tomatoes, diced

1 tablespoon Greek yogurt

Method:

Mix tuna, mashed avocado, diced tomatoes, and Greek yogurt.

Spoon into the avocado halves.

SPAGHETTI SQUASH AND MEATBALLS

Cooking Time: 20 minutes

Nutritional Benefits: Low-carb alternative with lean protein from turkey.

Ingredients:

1 cup cooked spaghetti squash

4 turkey meatballs

1/4 cup marinara sauce

Fresh basil for garnish

Method:

Heat turkey meatballs and marinara sauce.

Serve over spaghetti squash, garnish with fresh basil.

MEDITERRANEAN CHICKEN KEBABS

Cooking Time: 15 minutes

Nutritional Benefits: Protein-rich with a burst of Mediterranean flavors.

Ingredients:

4 oz chicken breast, cubed

Cherry tomatoes

Red onion, sliced

Zucchini, sliced

1 tablespoon olive oil

Lemon juice, to taste

Method:

Thread chicken, tomatoes, onion, and zucchini onto skewers.

Grill until chicken is cooked through.

Drizzle with olive oil and lemon juice before serving.

CAPRESE CHICKEN SALAD

Preparation Time: 10 minutes

Nutritional Benefits: High protein and healthy fats with a classic Caprese twist.

Ingredients:

4 oz grilled chicken breast, sliced

1 cup cherry tomatoes, halved

1/2 cup fresh mozzarella, diced

Fresh basil leaves

Balsamic glaze, for drizzling

Method:

Arrange sliced chicken, tomatoes, and mozzarella on a plate.

Garnish with fresh basil and drizzle with balsamic glaze.

VEGETABLE STIR-FRY WITH TOFU

Cooking Time: 15 minutes

Nutritional Benefits: Plant-based protein from tofu and a variety of veggies.

Ingredients:

1 cup broccoli florets

1/2 cup snap peas

1/2 cup tofu, cubcd

1/4 cup low-sodium soy sauce

1 tablespoon sesame oil

Method:

Sauté broccoli, snap peas, and tofu in sesame oil.

Drizzle with soy sauce and cook until vegetables are tender.

CAJUN SPICED SALMON BOWL

Cooking Time: 20 minutes

Nutritional Benefits: Omega-3s from salmon and a nutrient-packed grain bowl.

Ingredients:

4 oz Cajun-spiced salmon fillet

1/2 cup quinoa, cooked

1/4 cup black beans

1/4 cup corn kernels

Avocado slices for topping

Grill or bake salmon until cooked.

Arrange quinoa, black beans, corn, and top with salmon and avocado.

ROASTED VEGETABLE AND CHICKEN SALAD

Preparation Time: 15 minutes

Nutritional Benefits: Protein-packed salad with a variety of veggies.

Ingredients:

4 oz roasted chicken breast, shredded

Mixed greens

1/2 cup cherry tomatoes, halved

1/4 cup red bell peppers, sliced

1 tablespoon balsamic vinaigrette

Combine shredded chicken, mixed greens, tomatoes, and bell peppers.

Drizzle with balsamic vinaigrette.

LEMON HERB GRILLED TURKEY BURGERS

Cooking Time: 15 minutes

Nutritional Benefits: Lean protein from turkey with a burst of fresh flavors.

Ingredients:

4 oz ground turkey

1/2 teaspoon lemon zest

1/2 teaspoon dried herbs (such as thyme or oregano)

Lettuce leaves for wrapping

Sliced cucumber and tomato for topping

Method:

Mix ground turkey with lemon zest and dried herbs.

Form into patties and grill until cooked.

Serve wrapped in lettuce leaves with cucumber and tomato.

VEGETARIAN LENTIL SOUP

Cooking Time: 30 minutes
Nutritional Benefits: High in fiber and plant-based protein.

Ingredients:

1/2 cup dry lentils, rinsed

2 cups vegetable broth

1/2 cup diced carrots

1/2 cup diced celery

1/4 cup diced onion

Combine lentils, vegetable broth, carrots, celery, and onion in a pot.

Simmer until lentils are tender.

SWEET POTATO AND BLACK BEAN QUESADILLA

Cooking Time: 10 minutes

Nutritional Benefits: Fiber-rich and full of vitamins from sweet potatoes.

Ingredients:

1 small sweet potato, cooked and mashed

1/4 cup black beans, mashed

Whole-grain tortilla

1/4 cup shredded cheddar cheese

Method:

Spread mashed sweet potato and black beans on half of the tortilla.

Sprinkle with shredded cheddar, fold, and cook until cheese melts.

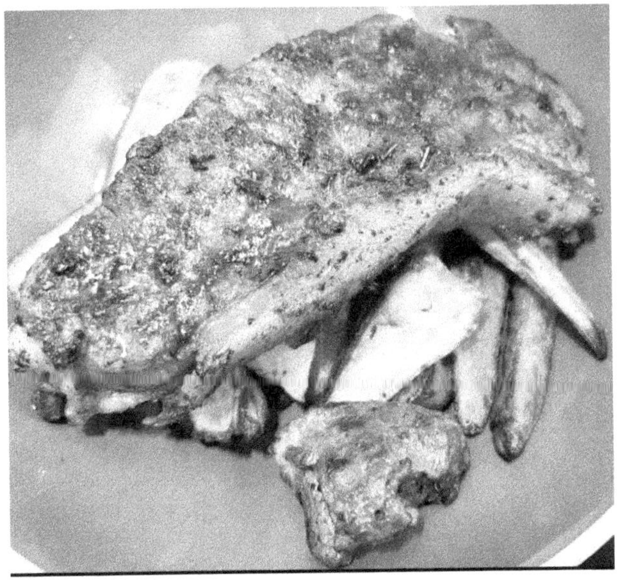

MANGO CHICKEN LETTUCE WRAPS

Preparation Time: 15 minutes

Nutritional Benefits: Lean protein from chicken with the natural sweetness of mango.

Ingredients:

4 oz grilled chicken breast, diced

Large lettuce leaves

1/2 cup diced mango

1/4 cup red bell peppers, sliced

Lime wedge for garnish

Method:

Fill lettuce leaves with diced chicken, mango, and bell peppers.

Squeeze lime juice before serving.

TURKEY AND VEGETABLE KABOBS

Cooking Time: 20 minutes

Nutritional Benefits: Lean protein with a mix of colorful veggies.

Ingredients:

4 oz turkey breast, cubed

Cherry tomatoes

Mushrooms, sliced

Red onion, sliced

1 tablespoon olive oil

Method:

Thread turkey, tomatoes, mushrooms, and onion onto skewers.

Grill until turkey is cooked, drizzle with olive oil.

CAULIFLOWER FRIED RICE WITH SHRIMP

Cooking Time: 15 minutes

Nutritional Benefits: Low-carb alternative with protein-packed shrimp.

Ingredients:

4 oz shrimp, peeled and deveined

1 cup cauliflower rice

1/4 cup peas and carrots, frozen

1/4 cup soy sauce

1 tablespoon sesame oil

Method:

Sauté shrimp, cauliflower rice, peas, and carrots in sesame oil.

Drizzle with soy sauce and cook until shrimp are pink.

GREEK YOGURT CHICKEN SALAD WRAP

Preparation Time: 10 minutes

Nutritional Benefits: Protein-rich and creamy with a hint of Mediterranean freshness.

Ingredients:

4 oz cooked chicken breast, shredded

Whole-grain wrap

2 tablespoons Greek yogurt

1/4 cup cucumber, diced

1/4 cup cherry tomatoes, halved

Method:

Mix shredded chicken with Greek yogurt, cucumber, and tomatoes.

Fill the wrap with the mixture.

SPICY BLACK BEAN AND VEGETABLE QUINOA BOWL

Cooking Time: 15 minutes

Nutritional Benefits: High in protein and fiber, packed with vitamins.

Ingredients:

1/2 cup cooked quinoa

1/4 cup black beans, cooked

1/2 cup diced bell peppers

1/4 cup corn kernels

1/4 teaspoon chili powder

Method:

Mix quinoa, black beans, bell peppers, corn, and chili powder.

Heat until warmed through.

CHICKEN AND AVOCADO LETTUCE WRAPS

Preparation Time: 15 minutes

Nutritional Benefits: Lean protein from chicken with the creamy goodness of avocado.

Ingredients:

4 oz grilled chicken breast, sliced

Large lettuce leaves

1/2 avocado, sliced

1/4 cup cherry tomatoes, halved

Cilantro for garnish

Method:

Arrange sliced chicken, avocado, and tomatoes on lettuce leaves.

Garnish with cilantro before serving.

MUSHROOM AND SPINACH STUFFED CHICKEN BREAST

Ingredients:

4 oz chicken breast

1/2 cup spinach, chopped

1/4 cup mushrooms, diced

1 tablespoon olive oil

Salt and pepper to taste

Method:

Preheat oven. Butterfly chicken breast.

Sauté spinach and mushrooms in olive oil, stuff into

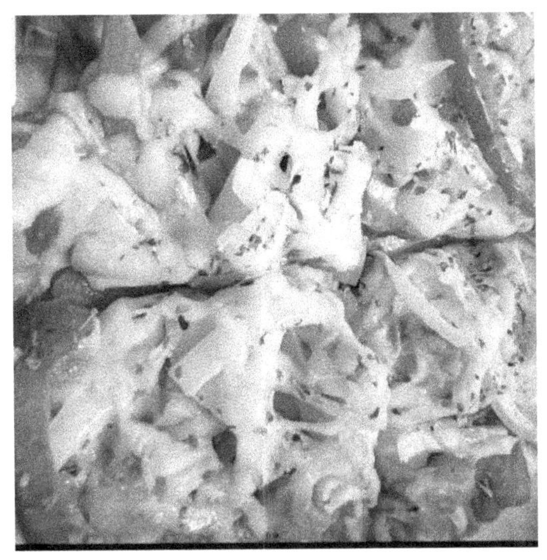

DINNER

GRILLED SALMON WITH LEMON DILL SAUCE

Cooking Time: 15 minutes

Nutritional Benefits: Omega-3 fatty acids from salmon, and antioxidants from lemon and dill.

Ingredients:

6 oz salmon fillet

1 tablespoon olive oil

1 teaspoon lemon zest

1 tablespoon fresh dill, chopped

Method:

Rub salmon with olive oil, lemon zest, and dill.

Grill until salmon is cooked through.

CAULIFLOWER AND BROCCOLI ALFREDO

Cooking Time: 20 minutes
Nutritional Benefits: Low-calorie, low-carb, and high in vitamins and fiber.

Ingredients:

1 cup cauliflower, steamed

1 cup broccoli florets, steamed

1/2 cup unsweetened almond milk

2 tablespoons nutritional yeast

1 clove garlic, minced

Method:

Blend cauliflower, broccoli, almond milk, nutritional yeast, and garlic until smooth.

Heat and pour over your favorite protein or low-carb pasta.

LEMON GARLIC CHICKEN STIR-FRY

Cooking Time: 15 minutes

Nutritional Benefits: Lean protein from chicken, vitamin C from bell peppers, and antioxidants from lemon.

Ingredients:

4 oz chicken breast, sliced

1 cup broccoli florets

1/2 bell pepper, sliced

1 tablespoon olive oil

1 teaspoon lemon juice

Method:

Sauté chicken, broccoli, and bell pepper in olive oil.

Drizzle with lemon juice before serving.

SPAGHETTI SQUASH WITH TURKEY BOLOGNESE

Cooking Time: 30 minutes

Nutritional Benefits: Low-carb alternative with lean protein and vitamins.

Ingredients:

1 medium spaghetti squash, cooked and shredded

4 oz ground turkey

1/2 cup tomato sauce

1 clove garlic, minced

1/2 teaspoon Italian seasoning

Method:

Sauté ground turkey, add garlic, tomato sauce, and seasoning.

Serve over shredded spaghetti squash.

ASIAN INSPIRED VEGGIE AND TOFU STIR-FRY

Cooking Time: 20 minutes

Nutritional Benefits: Plant-based protein from tofu and a variety of veggies.

Ingredients:

1 cup tofu, cubed

1 cup broccoli florets

1/2 cup snap peas

1/4 cup low-sodium soy sauce

1 tablespoon sesame oil

Sauté tofu, broccoli, and snap peas in sesame oil.

Drizzle with soy sauce and cook until vegetables are tender.

TURKEY AND BLACK BEAN CHILI

Cooking Time: 25 minutes

Nutritional Benefits: Lean protein from turkey, fiber from black beans, and antioxidants from tomatoes.

Ingredients:

4 oz ground turkey

1/2 cup black beans, cooked

1/2 cup diced tomatoes

1 teaspoon chili powder

1/4 cup chopped cilantro for garnish

Method:

Sauté ground turkey, add black beans, tomatoes, and chili powder.

Simmer until flavors meld. Garnish with cilantro.

ROASTED BRUSSELS SPROUTS AND CHICKEN THIGHS

Cooking Time: 30 minutes

Nutritional Benefits: Protein from chicken thighs and fiber from Brussels sprouts.

Ingredients:

4 oz chicken thighs, skin-on

1 cup Brussels sprouts, halved

1 tablespoon olive oil

Salt and pepper to taste

Method:

Rub chicken with olive oil, season with salt and pepper.

Roast chicken and Brussels sprouts until golden and cooked through.

EGGPLANT LASAGNA

Cooking Time: 30 minutes

Nutritional Benefits: Low-carb, high-fiber alternative to traditional lasagna.

Ingredients:

1 large eggplant, sliced

1 cup ricotta cheese

1/2 cup marinara sauce

1/4 cup grated Parmesan cheese

Grill or bake eggplant slices until tender.

Layer with ricotta, marinara, and Parmesan. Bake until bubbly.

MISO GLAZED SALMON WITH QUINOA

Cooking Time: 20 minutes

Nutritional Benefits: Omega-3s from salmon and a protein-packed grain.

Ingredients:

6 oz salmon fillet

2 tablespoons miso paste

1 tablespoon soy sauce

1 cup cooked quinoa

Method:

Mix miso paste and soy sauce. Coat salmon and bake until flaky.

Serve over a bed of cooked quinoa.

CAJUN SPICED CHICKEN WITH CAULIFLOWER MASH

Cooking Time: 25 minutes

Nutritional Benefits: Lean protein from chicken, low-carb mashed cauliflower.

Ingredients:

4 oz chicken breast

1 teaspoon Cajun seasoning

1 cup cauliflower, steamed and mashed

1 tablespoon olive oil

Method:

Rub chicken with Cajun seasoning, cook until done.

Serve over a bed of cauliflower mash drizzled with olive oil.

GARLIC HERB TURKEY MEATBALLS WITH ZOODLES

Cooking Time: 20 minutes
Nutritional Benefits: Lean protein from turkey, low-carb zoodles, and antioxidant-rich herbs.

Ingredients:

4 oz ground turkey

1 clove garlic, minced

1 tablespoon fresh herbs (parsley, basil), chopped

1 zucchini, spiralized

1/4 cup marinara sauce

Method:

Mix ground turkey with garlic and herbs. Form into meatballs.

Bake until cooked through. Serve over zoodles with marinara sauce.

SPINACH AND FETA STUFFED CHICKEN BREAST

Cooking Time: 25 minutes

Nutritional Benefits: Lean protein from chicken, iron-rich spinach, and calcium from feta.

Ingredients:

4 oz chicken breast

1 cup fresh spinach

2 tablespoons feta cheese

1/2 teaspoon lemon zest

Method:

Butterfly chicken breast. Stuff with spinach, feta, and lemon zest.

Bake until chicken is cooked through.

BROCCOLI AND CHEDDAR STUFFED PEPPERS

Cooking Time: 20 minutes

Nutritional Benefits: Fiber from bell peppers, calcium from cheddar, and protein from Greek yogurt.

Ingredients:

2 bell peppers, halved

1 cup broccoli florets, steamed

1/2 cup shredded cheddar cheese

1/4 cup Greek yogurt

Method:

Steam broccoli and mix with cheddar and Greek yogurt.

Stuff bell peppers and bake until cheese is melted.

TANDOORI CHICKEN SKEWERS WITH CUCUMBER RAITA

Cooking Time: 15 minutes

Nutritional Benefits: Lean protein from chicken, probiotics from yogurt, and antioxidants from mint.

Ingredients:

4 oz chicken breast, cubed

1 tablespoon tandoori spice blend

1/2 cup cucumber, diced

1/4 cup plain yogurt

Fresh mint for garnish

Method:

Coat chicken with tandoori spice. Skewer and grill until cooked.

Mix cucumber with yogurt for raita. Garnish with fresh mint.

CAPRESE ZUCCHINI NOODLE BOWL

Cooking Time: 10 minutes

Nutritional Benefits: Low-carb, high-fiber, and a burst of flavor with tomatoes and basil.

Ingredients:

1 zucchini, spiralized

1/2 cup cherry tomatoes, halved

1/4 cup fresh mozzarella, diced

Fresh basil leaves

Balsamic glaze for drizzling

Sauté zoodles until tender. Top with tomatoes, mozzarella, and basil.

Drizzle with balsamic glaze before serving.

SHRIMP AND AVOCADO CEVICHE

Preparation Time: 15 minutes

Nutritional Benefits: Lean protein from shrimp, healthy fats from avocado, and vitamin C from lime.

Ingredients:

4 oz shrimp, cooked and diced

1/2 avocado, diced

1/4 cup red onion, finely chopped

1/4 cup cilantro, chopped

Lime juice to taste

Method:

Combine shrimp, avocado, red onion, and cilantro.

Squeeze lime juice, toss, and refrigerate before serving.

MEDITERRANEAN STUFFED ZUCCHINI BOATS

Cooking Time: 25 minutes

Nutritional Benefits: Fiber-rich and high in vitamins and minerals.

Ingredients:

2 zucchinis, halved

1/2 cup cooked quinoa

1/4 cup Kalamata olives, chopped

1/4 cup cherry tomatoes, diced

Feta cheese for topping

Method:

Scoop out zucchini centers. Mix quinoa, olives, and tomatoes.

Stuff zucchini halves, top with feta, and bake until zucchini is tender.

THAI BASIL CHICKEN STIR-FRY

Cooking Time: 15 minutes

Nutritional Benefits: Lean protein from chicken and a variety of veggies with a Thai-inspired twist.

Ingredients:

4 oz chicken breast, sliced

1 cup bell peppers, sliced

1/2 cup snap peas

1 tablespoon soy sauce

Fresh basil leaves for garnish

Method:

Sauté chicken, bell peppers, and snap peas in soy sauce.

Garnish with fresh basil before serving.

LEMON HERB ROASTED CHICKEN THIGHS

Cooking Time: 30 minutes

Nutritional Benefits: Protein from chicken thighs with a burst of citrusy flavor.

Ingredients:

4 oz chicken thighs, skin-on

1 lemon, sliced

1 tablespoon olive oil

1 teaspoon dried herbs (rosemary, thyme)

Method:

Preheat oven. Rub chicken with olive oil and herbs.

Place lemon slices on top and roast until chicken is golden and cooked.

CAULIFLOWER AND SPINACH GRATIN

Ingredients:

1 cup cauliflower, steamed and chopped

1 cup fresh spinach, chopped

1/2 cup shredded cheddar cheese

1/4 cup heavy cream

Method:

Mix cauliflower, spinach, cheddar, and heavy cream.

Bake until the top is golden and bubbly.

CONCLUSION

As we enjoy the last few chapters of our gastric bypass cookbook, we find ourselves engulfed in the rich tapestry of flavors, nutrients, and just learned culinary wisdom has imparted. This cookbook has been more than simply a recipe book; it's been a friend, a mentor, and a celebration of the road to goodness, recovery, and well-being.

With each meticulously crafted dish, we've studied the art of cooking meals that specifically meet the needs of gastric health, finding a balance between the need for nourishment and the need for indulgence that satisfies the palate. From soothing soups to inventive major meals, the "Gastric Bypass Cookbook" has transported us to a world of gastronomic delights tailored to people looking for a conscientious and health-conscious approach to dining.

As you embark on your own culinary adventure, may the knowledge contained inside these pages serve as a guide, adding happiness and nourishment to each dish you prepare. Take advantage of this opportunity to nourish your body and soul, but remember that cooking for stomach health is a powerful experience that requires creativity and attention to detail.

To everyone aspiring to be gourmet chefs: may your kitchens be filled with the aromas of wholesome foods and may your meals be a well-balanced fusion of flavors that enhance well-being. I hope that as you experiment with these recipes and add your own special touch, you will have a newfound appreciation for the healing power of food.

I wish you vibrant health, delectable meals, and many years of delighting in the satisfaction of giving your body the most exquisite sustenance imaginable. Cheers to your culinary journey and the fascinating world of the "Gastric Bypass Cookbook"! Let's toast to a delicious meal that can transform you into a more positive, self-aware person.